# Resistance Band Exercise Guide for Beginners

## Embracing a Sustainable Fitness Routine

By

Latharn Naois

# Table of Contents

# CHAPTER 1

# Introduction

## 1.1 What Are Resistance Bands?

Resistance bands, also known as exercise bands or workout bands, are versatile and flexible tools used in strength training and physical fitness. These bands are typically made of latex or other elastic materials and come in various shapes, sizes, and resistance levels. They're often color-coded to signify different levels of resistance, allowing individuals to progressively increase the intensity of their exercises as they get stronger.

Resistance bands work on a simple principle: they create tension in the form of resistance when stretched. This resistance challenges your muscles, making them work harder during exercises. The level of resistance varies depending on the band's thickness, length, and the material used in its construction.

These bands are incredibly adaptable and can be incorporated into a wide range of exercises, targeting various muscle groups in your body. You can use resistance bands for both upper body and lower body workouts, making them a versatile choice for anyone looking to improve their strength and overall fitness.

## 1.2 Benefits of Using Resistance Bands

Using resistance bands offers a multitude of benefits that make them an attractive option for people of all fitness levels. Here, we'll delve into some of the primary advantages:

**1. Improved Strength and Muscle Tone:** Resistance bands provide an effective means of building and toning muscles. As you perform exercises with these bands, your muscles must exert force to overcome the resistance. Over time, this leads to increased muscle strength and definition. What's great is that resistance bands are accommodating for beginners and advanced users alike, allowing you to start at your fitness level and progress from there.

**2. Portability and Convenience:**
Resistance bands are incredibly portable and can be taken anywhere, making them a convenient choice for people with busy schedules or those who travel frequently. You can easily toss a resistance band in your bag, and it won't take up much space. This convenience means you can fit in a workout virtually anywhere, whether you're at home, in a hotel room, or outdoors.

**3. Joint-Friendly Workouts:** Unlike some traditional weightlifting exercises, resistance band exercises are generally low-impact. This makes them gentler on your joints, which can be particularly beneficial for individuals with joint issues or those recovering from injuries. The consistent tension applied by resistance bands also promotes stability and joint health.

**4. Versatility:** Resistance bands are incredibly versatile and can be used to target virtually every muscle group in your body. You can perform a wide range of exercises, from bicep curls and tricep extensions to squats, lunges, and even core exercises. This versatility allows you to create a well-rounded workout routine that addresses your specific fitness goals.

**5. Adaptability for All Fitness Levels:** One of the most significant advantages of resistance bands is their adaptability. You can easily adjust the resistance level by using different bands or altering your body's position relative to the band. This means that whether you're a beginner or an experienced athlete, resistance bands can be tailored to your needs and capabilities.

**6. Affordable and Cost-Effective:** Resistance bands are an economical fitness solution when compared to the cost of purchasing traditional gym equipment or a gym membership. They offer a cost-effective way to maintain or improve your fitness without breaking the bank.

**7. Improved Balance and Coordination:** Resistance bands require stabilization, as they often don't offer the same stability as machines or free weights. This means that when you incorporate them into your workouts, you're not only building strength but also enhancing your balance and coordination.

resistance bands are simple yet effective tools that can play a significant role in helping beginners kickstart their fitness journey. Their flexibility, portability, and ability to provide a comprehensive full-body workout make them a fantastic choice for those seeking to improve their strength and overall well-being. As you progress through this guide, you'll discover various resistance band exercises and workouts tailored for beginners, helping you unlock the many benefits these bands have to offer.

# CHAPTER 2
# Getting Started

## 2.1 Choosing the Right Resistance Band

Selecting the appropriate resistance band is a crucial step in your journey to harness the benefits of resistance band exercises. The right band ensures that your workouts are both challenging and safe. Here, we'll delve into the factors you should consider when choosing a resistance band:

- **Resistance Level:** Resistance bands come in different resistance levels, typically denoted by colors or labels such as "light," "medium," or "heavy." As a beginner, it's essential to start with a lighter resistance band and gradually progress to higher levels as your strength improves.

- **Material:** Resistance bands are often made from latex or other elastic materials. Consider any allergies or sensitivities you might have when choosing the material. Some bands are latex-free to accommodate those with latex allergies.

- **Length and Thickness:** The length and thickness of the band can impact the resistance it provides. Longer bands generally offer more resistance, and thicker bands are typically harder to stretch. As a beginner, it's advisable to start with a medium-length and thickness band for versatility.

- **Handles or Loops:** Some resistance bands come with handles or loops for better grip and versatility in exercises. Depending on your preference and the types of exercises you plan to do, you may choose a band with or without handles.

- **Ankle Straps:** If you plan to use resistance bands for lower body exercises, look for bands that come with ankle straps. These straps attach to the band and allow you to secure it around your ankles for exercises like leg lifts and glute work.

- **Quality:** Ensure that the resistance band is of good

quality and durability. You want a band that can withstand stretching and repeated use without snapping or losing its elasticity.

your choice of resistance band should match your current fitness level and the specific exercises you plan to perform. Starting with a lighter resistance band and gradually progressing as you become stronger is the safest and most effective approach.

## 2.2 Safety Precautions and Tips

Safety is paramount when using resistance bands, as with any form of exercise. Here are some essential safety precautions and tips to keep in mind:

- **Inspect Your Band:** Before each use, inspect your resistance band for any signs of wear and tear. Check for cuts, cracks, or any visible damage. A damaged band should not be used, as it can snap during exercise, potentially causing injury.

- **Secure Anchoring:** When attaching a resistance band to an anchor point (e.g., a door handle or sturdy object), ensure it's secure and won't come loose during your workout. A loose attachment can lead to accidents.

- **Maintain Proper Form:** Correct form is crucial for

effective and safe resistance band exercises. Pay attention to your posture and positioning to prevent straining or injuring your muscles.

- **Start Slow:** If you're new to resistance band exercises, begin with simple and low-resistance movements. Gradually increase the intensity as your muscles adapt and become stronger.

- **Control the Band:** Maintain control of the resistance band throughout the entire range of motion during exercises. Letting the band snap back uncontrollably can lead to accidents.

- **Warm-Up:** Always warm up your muscles before engaging in resistance band workouts. A brief warm-up can help reduce the risk of injury.

- **Consult a Professional:** If you have any existing medical conditions or are unsure about which exercises are suitable for your fitness level, it's advisable to consult a fitness professional or a physical therapist for guidance.

Following these safety precautions and tips, you can ensure that your resistance band workouts are not only effective but also safe.

## 2.3 Setting Up Your Workout Space

Creating a conducive workout space is essential for a productive and injury-free resistance band exercise

session. Here's how to set up your
workout space:

- **Clear the Area:** Ensure that
  the area where you plan to
  work out is free from clutter
  and hazards. Remove any
  objects that could cause
  tripping or falling.

- **Anchor Point:** If you're using
  resistance bands that require
  anchoring, select a sturdy
  anchor point. This could be a
  closed door (using a door
  anchor), a secure wall mount,
  or a heavy piece of furniture.

- **Flooring:** Opt for a non-slip
  and cushioned surface, such as
  a yoga mat or exercise mat, to
  prevent slipping and provide a
  bit of shock absorption.

- **Ample Space:** Make sure you have enough space to perform your exercises without restriction. Most resistance band exercises don't require a large area, but having room to move comfortably is essential.

- **Lighting and Ventilation:** Adequate lighting is important to see your surroundings and maintain proper form. Good ventilation helps you stay cool and comfortable during your workout.

- **Mirror (Optional):** If available, positioning a mirror in your workout space can help you monitor your form and ensure you're performing exercises correctly.

- **Music or Entertainment:** Many people find that playing music or having a fitness video on hand can make their workouts more enjoyable and motivating. Prepare any entertainment you prefer in advance.

Setting up your workout space thoughtfully, you'll create an environment that supports your resistance band exercises and contributes to a safe and enjoyable fitness routine.

# CHAPTER 3

# Basic Resistance Band Exercises

## 3.1 Bicep Curls

Bicep curls are a fundamental resistance band exercise that targets the biceps, the muscles in the front of your upper arm. Here's how to perform bicep curls with a resistance band:

1. Stand with both feet on the center of the resistance band, holding one end in each hand, palms facing forward.

2. Keep your back straight, core engaged, and elbows close to your torso.

3.  Slowly curl your hands upward towards your shoulders while keeping your upper arms stationary. Squeeze your biceps at the top of the movement.

4.  Lower your hands back down to the starting position in a controlled manner.

5.  Repeat for the desired number of repetitions.

Bicep curls are an excellent way to build strength and definition in your biceps, and with resistance bands, you can easily adjust the intensity by using bands with different levels of resistance.

## 3.2 Tricep Extensions

Tricep extensions with resistance bands are an effective way to target the triceps, the muscles on the back of your upper arms. Here's how to perform tricep extensions:

1. Stand on the center of the resistance band with your feet hip-width apart. Hold one end of the band in each hand, with your palms facing up and your arms extended overhead.

2. Keep your core engaged and your back straight.

3. Bend your elbows and lower your hands behind your head, keeping your upper arms stationary.

4. Straighten your arms, extending them fully overhead, and squeeze your triceps at the top of the movement.

5.  Lower your hands back down behind your head in a controlled manner.

6.  Repeat for the desired number of repetitions.

Tricep extensions are a great way to strengthen and tone your triceps, and they can be adjusted in difficulty by using bands with different resistance levels.

# 3.3 Bent-Over Rows

Bent-over rows are a versatile resistance band exercise that primarily targets the muscles of your upper back, including the latissimus dorsi. Here's how to perform bent-over rows:

1.  Stand on the center of the resistance band with your feet

shoulder-width apart. Hold one end of the band in each hand, palms facing each other, and let the band hang in front of you.

2. Hinge at your hips, keeping your back flat and your knees slightly bent. Your upper body should be inclined forward at about a 45-degree angle.

3. Engage your core and pull the band towards your lower ribs by bending your elbows and squeezing your shoulder blades together.

4. Slowly return the band to the starting position, fully extending your arms.

5. Repeat for the desired number of repetitions.

Bent-over rows are an effective exercise for developing upper body strength, especially in the back and shoulder muscles. Using resistance bands allows you to adjust the challenge by using bands with different resistance levels.

## 3.4 Squats

Squats with resistance bands are a compound exercise that primarily targets the muscles in your lower body, including the quadriceps, hamstrings, and glutes. Here's how to perform squats with a resistance band:

1. Step onto the center of the resistance band with your feet shoulder-width apart, positioning your feet evenly on the band.

2.  Hold one end of the band in each hand, and bring your hands up to your shoulders, so your palms are facing forward.

3.  Engage your core, keep your back straight, and maintain an upright posture.

4.  Begin the squat by bending at your hips and knees, as if you're sitting back into an imaginary chair. Keep your knees aligned with your toes.

5.  Lower your body until your thighs are parallel to the ground or as far as your flexibility allows.

6.  Push through your heels to stand back up to the starting position, fully extending your legs.

7. Repeat for the desired number of repetitions.

Squats with resistance bands are an excellent exercise for building lower body strength and enhancing overall leg muscle tone. The resistance band adds an extra challenge to the movement, making it more effective in building muscle and strength.

# 3.5 Standing Chest Press

The standing chest press with a resistance band is a versatile exercise that targets the chest and front shoulder muscles. Here's how to perform the standing chest press:

1. Anchor the resistance band securely at chest height, using a door anchor or another stable point.

2. Stand facing away from the anchor point, holding one end of the band in each hand.

3. Extend your arms forward at chest level, with your palms facing down.

4. Stand with one foot slightly in front of the other for balance.

5. Engage your core and maintain an upright posture.

6. Push the bands away from your chest, fully extending your arms.

7. Slowly return your hands to the starting position in a controlled manner.

8. Repeat for the desired number of repetitions.

The standing chest press is an effective exercise for targeting the chest and front shoulders, and the resistance band allows for adjustable resistance levels.

## 3.6 Leg Lifts

Leg lifts with resistance bands are a great exercise for targeting your lower abdominal muscles. Here's how to perform leg lifts using a resistance band:

1.  Lie on your back on a mat with your legs extended.

2.  Anchor the resistance band around the bottom of a sturdy object, such as a table leg or a heavy piece of furniture.

3.  Loop the other end of the band around your ankles, securing it in place.

4.  Place your hands under your hips or hold onto the sides of the mat for stability.

5.  Engage your core and lift your legs off the ground, keeping them straight.

6.  Lift your legs as high as you can while maintaining control and without arching your back excessively.

7.  Slowly lower your legs back down, almost touching the ground but not resting them completely.

8.  Repeat for the desired number of repetitions.

Leg lifts with a resistance band effectively engage the lower abdominal muscles, providing a challenging workout for your core.

## 3.7 Glute Bridges

Glute bridges with a resistance band are an excellent exercise for strengthening the glutes and hamstrings. Here's how to perform glute bridges using a resistance band:

1.  Lie on your back on a mat with your knees bent and feet flat on the ground.

2.  Place the resistance band just above your knees, and make sure it's secure.

3.  Place your arms by your sides with your palms facing down.

4.  Engage your core, and press your heels into the ground to lift your hips off the mat.

5.  Squeeze your glutes at the top of the movement, creating a straight line from your shoulders to your knees.

6.  Hold the bridge position briefly at the top.

7.  Lower your hips back down to the mat in a controlled manner.

8.  Repeat for the desired number of repetitions.

Glute bridges with a resistance band are effective for targeting and strengthening the glute muscles while also engaging the hamstrings. The resistance band adds an extra challenge to the exercise by activating the glutes more intensely.

# CHAPTER 4

# Sample Resistance Band Workouts

## 4.1 Full-Body Resistance Band Workout

A full-body resistance band workout is an excellent way to engage all major muscle groups in a single session. This workout is designed to provide a comprehensive training experience. Remember to choose resistance bands that match your fitness level. Perform each exercise for 10-15 repetitions and aim for 2-3 sets.

**Warm-Up:**

- Jumping jacks or jogging in place for 5 minutes to raise your heart rate and warm up your muscles.

**Workout:**

1. **Squats with Resistance Band**

   - Targets: Quads, hamstrings, glutes, and calves.

2. **Bicep Curls**

   - Targets: Biceps.

3. **Tricep Extensions**

   - Targets: Triceps.

4. **Bent-Over Rows**

   - Targets: Upper back, lats, and rear shoulders.

5. **Standing Chest Press**

- Targets: Chest and front shoulders.

6. **Leg Lifts (Using a Door Anchor)**

   - Targets: Lower abdominals.

7. **Glute Bridges**

   - Targets: Glutes and hamstrings.

8. **Plank with Shoulder Taps**

   - Targets: Core, shoulders, and upper body stability.

**Cool Down:**

- Stretch all major muscle groups, holding each stretch for 15-30 seconds. Focus on the legs, arms, chest, back, and shoulders.

This full-body resistance band workout provides a well-rounded training experience, helping you build strength and tone various muscle groups in your body.

## 4.2 Upper Body Workout

An upper body resistance band workout focuses on strengthening the muscles of the arms, shoulders, and back. As with any workout, choose resistance bands that suit your fitness level. Perform each exercise for 10-15 repetitions and aim for 2-3 sets.

**Warm-Up:**

- Arm circles and shoulder rolls for 3-5 minutes to warm up the upper body.

**Workout:**

1. **Bicep Curls**

   - Targets: Biceps.

2. **Tricep Extensions**

   - Targets: Triceps.

3. **Standing Chest Press**

   - Targets: Chest and front shoulders.

4. **Bent-Over Rows**

   - Targets: Upper back, lats, and rear shoulders.

5. **Lateral Raises**

   - Targets: Side shoulders.

6. **Front Raises**

   - Targets: Front shoulders.

7. **Push-Ups with Resistance Band (optional)**

- Targets: Chest, triceps, and shoulders.

8. **Arm Pull-Aparts**

   - Targets: Rear shoulders and upper back.

**Cool Down:**

- Stretch the arms, shoulders, and upper back. Hold each stretch for 15-30 seconds, focusing on the muscles worked during the workout.

This upper body resistance band workout will help you build strength, improve muscle definition, and enhance upper body stability. It's a fantastic option for those looking to focus on their upper body strength and fitness.

# 4.3 Lower Body Workout

A lower body resistance band workout is designed to target the muscles in your legs and buttocks. It's an effective way to strengthen and tone the lower body while improving overall lower body stability. As always, choose resistance bands that match your fitness level. Perform each exercise for 10-15 repetitions and aim for 2-3 sets.

**Warm-Up:**

- Leg swings and dynamic stretches for 5 minutes to warm up the lower body.

**Workout:**

1. **Squats with Resistance Band**

    - Targets: Quads, hamstrings, glutes, and calves.

2.  **Lunges (Forward and Reverse)**

  - Targets: Quads, hamstrings, glutes, and calves.

3.  **Leg Lifts (Using a Door Anchor)**

  - Targets: Lower abdominals.

4.  **Glute Bridges**

  - Targets: Glutes and hamstrings.

5.  **Clamshells**

  - Targets: Gluteus medius (the muscle on the side of your buttocks).

6.  **Fire Hydrants**

- Targets: Gluteus
  maximus (the large
  buttocks muscle).

7. **Side Leg Raises**

   - Targets: Outer thighs
     (abductors).

8. **Standing Calf Raises**

   - Targets: Calves.

**Cool Down:**

- Stretch the legs and lower body
  muscles. Focus on the quads,
  hamstrings, calves, and glutes,
  holding each stretch for 15-30
  seconds.

This lower body resistance band
workout is a fantastic way to
strengthen and tone your leg muscles
and enhance lower body stability. It's
suitable for individuals looking to

target and improve the strength and appearance of their lower body.

## 4.4 Core Strengthening Routine

A core strengthening routine with resistance bands is an effective way to target your abdominal muscles and lower back while also engaging your obliques and improving overall core stability. Choose resistance bands that match your fitness level. Perform each exercise for 10-15 repetitions and aim for 2-3 sets.

**Warm-Up:**

- Perform dynamic stretches or light core activation exercises, such as torso twists and leg lifts, for 5 minutes.

**Workout:**

1.  **Plank with Shoulder Taps**

    - Targets: Core, shoulders, and upper body stability.

2.  **Russian Twists**

    - Targets: Obliques and core.

3.  **Bicycle Crunches (Using a Door Anchor)**

    - Targets: Abdominals and obliques.

4.  **Woodchoppers**

    - Targets: Obliques and core.

5.  **Bird Dogs**

    - Targets: Lower back and core.

6. **Seated Leg Raises (With Band Around Feet)**

   - Targets: Lower abdominals.

7. **Supermans (With Band Around Wrists)**

   - Targets: Lower back and core.

8. **Standing Anti-Rotation Twists**

   - Targets: Obliques and core stability.

**Cool Down:**

- Stretch your core and lower back, holding each stretch for 15-30 seconds. Focus on stretching your abdominals, lower back, and obliques.

This core strengthening routine with resistance bands will help you build a strong and stable core, improve posture, and reduce the risk of lower back pain. It's a valuable addition to your fitness routine, promoting a balanced and well-conditioned core.

# CHAPTER 5

# Progression and Variation

## 5.1 Increasing Resistance

As you advance in your resistance band workouts, it's essential to continuously challenge your muscles to promote growth and strength development. Increasing resistance is a key component of progression. Here are some strategies for increasing resistance in your workouts:

1. **Switch to a Heavier Band:** The most straightforward way to increase resistance is to use a resistance band with a higher

resistance level. Many resistance bands come in different colors or with labels indicating their resistance levels. Gradually transition to a band with more resistance as your strength improves.

2. **Double Up the Bands:** To create even more resistance, you can double up on bands. Loop two or more bands together, or stand on multiple bands to increase the overall tension. Be cautious with this method and ensure the bands are securely attached to prevent snapping.

3. **Extend the Band:** You can make the band feel more challenging by increasing its length. Instead of standing directly on the band for

exercises, step on it with a wider stance, creating more tension when you stretch the band.

4. **Slow Down the Repetitions:** Slowing down the speed of your repetitions can make the exercises more challenging. This approach requires more muscle control and time under tension, which can lead to greater strength gains.

5. **Increase the Number of Repetitions and Sets:** As your strength improves, you can increase the number of repetitions or sets you perform for each exercise. Gradually progress from 10-15 reps to 15-20 or more, or from 2-3 sets to 4 or 5.

6. **Incorporate Isometric Holds:**
   Add isometric holds to your
   exercises. Pause at the most
   challenging part of an exercise
   (e.g., the top of a bicep curl)
   and hold for a few seconds
   before completing the
   repetition. Isometric holds
   intensify the exercise and
   promote strength gains.

7. **Change the Band's Anchor
   Point:** Adjust the anchor point
   of the band to change the angle
   and resistance during exercises.
   This can provide a different
   challenge and work your
   muscles from different angles.

8. **Use Resistance Band
   Accessories:** Some resistance
   band accessories, like handles,
   ankle straps, or door anchors,
   can allow for a wider range of

exercises and create more resistance options.

9. **Combine Exercises:** Combine different exercises to create more complex movements. For example, you can combine a squat with a shoulder press to target multiple muscle groups simultaneously.

10. **Progressive Overload:** The principle of progressive overload involves gradually increasing the resistance or intensity of your workouts over time. This is a fundamental concept in strength training and ensures continued improvement.

Progression should be gradual and tailored to your fitness level. Overloading too quickly can lead to overuse injuries. Keep track of your progress, listen to your body, and make adjustments as needed to ensure safe and effective progression in your resistance band workouts.

## 5.2 Combining Exercises

Combining exercises with resistance bands is a creative way to add variety to your workouts and target multiple muscle groups in a single routine. This can make your workouts more efficient and engaging. Here are some ideas for combining exercises with resistance bands:

1. **Squat to Overhead Press:** Combine squats and overhead presses for a full-body workout. Stand on the resistance band, hold the handles at shoulder height, and perform a squat. As

you stand up from the squat, press the bands overhead.

2. **Lunges with Rows:** Incorporate lunges with bent-over rows to work your legs and back simultaneously. Step on the band with one foot and perform lunges while holding the band handles. As you lunge forward, perform a rowing motion by pulling the handles toward your torso.

3. **Push-Up with Leg Lift:** Add leg lifts to your push-ups for an extra core and glute workout. Secure the band around your ankles and perform push-ups while lifting one leg off the ground at the top of each push-up.

4.  **Plank to Row:** Strengthen your core and upper body by combining planks and rows. Attach the band to an anchor point at chest height, get into a plank position, and row the band towards your chest.

5.  **Deadlift to Upright Row:** Combine deadlifts with upright rows to target your lower back and shoulders. Stand on the band with your feet hip-width apart, hold the handles in front of you, and perform a deadlift. As you stand up, transition into an upright row.

6.  **Squat to Lateral Leg Lift:** Enhance your leg and glute workout by adding lateral leg lifts to squats. Step on the band with both feet, perform a squat, and lift one leg to the side as

you return to the standing
position.

7. **Plank with Knee to Elbow:**
Create a challenging core
workout by performing planks
and bringing your knees to your
elbows. Attach the band to an
anchor point, get into a plank
position, and bring your knees
towards your elbows while
maintaining the plank.

8. **Bicep Curl to Tricep
Extension:** Work both your
biceps and triceps by
combining bicep curls with
tricep extensions. Stand on the
band, hold the handles, and
perform a bicep curl. After the
curl, transition into a tricep
extension.

9.  **Squat with Lateral Raise:**
Engage your legs and shoulders
by incorporating squats with
lateral raises. Stand on the
band, hold the handles at your
sides, and perform a squat. As
you stand up, raise your arms to
the sides.

10. **Push-Up with Shoulder Tap:**
Combine push-ups with
shoulder taps to target your
chest and shoulders while
improving core stability. Secure
the band around your wrists,
get into a push-up position, and
tap one shoulder with the
opposite hand between push-
ups.

Combining exercises not only adds
variety to your routine but also
challenges your muscles in new ways,
making your workouts more effective

and interesting. Ensure that you maintain proper form and alignment during these combined exercises to maximize their benefits and minimize the risk of injury.

## 5.3 Advanced Resistance Band Techniques

Advanced resistance band techniques are designed for individuals who have developed strength and coordination through regular resistance band workouts. These techniques can help you take your training to the next level and introduce greater complexity and challenge. Before attempting advanced techniques, ensure that you have mastered the basic exercises and have good form. Here are some advanced resistance band techniques:

1.  **Pause Repetitions:** Incorporate pauses in different parts of an exercise. For example, in a squat, pause at the bottom of the movement before returning to the starting position. This technique increases time under tension and muscle engagement.

2.  **Negative Repetitions:** Focus on the eccentric phase of an exercise, which is the lowering phase. For instance, during a bicep curl, emphasize the controlled lowering of the resistance band rather than the lifting phase. This technique is excellent for building muscle strength.

3.  **Band Resisted Plyometrics:** Integrate resistance bands into plyometric exercises like jump

squats, box jumps, or burpees. The bands add extra resistance to explosive movements, making them more challenging and effective for power development.

4. **Partial Range of Motion (ROM) Exercises:** Concentrate on a specific portion of an exercise's range of motion. For example, perform half-range squats or half-range push-ups. This technique targets different muscle fibers and can break plateaus in your training.

5. **Drop Sets:** Combine resistance bands with a variety of bands of different resistance levels. Start with the heaviest band for an exercise, and as you reach failure, switch to a lighter band to continue the set. This

technique can lead to muscle fatigue and growth.

6. **Supersets and Giant Sets:** String together multiple exercises with minimal rest in between. For instance, perform a set of bicep curls, followed immediately by tricep extensions, then bent-over rows, with minimal rest in between. This technique is excellent for enhancing muscle endurance.

7. **Isometric Holds with Bands:** Add isometric holds to exercises by pausing at the most challenging part of the movement and holding it for several seconds. For example, during a leg lift, pause at the highest point and hold. This

technique promotes muscle
endurance and engagement.

8.  **Resistance Band Drop Sets:**
    Use a single band but fold it in
    half or more to create increased
    resistance as you progress
    through a set. As you fatigue,
    unfold the band to decrease
    resistance and continue the set.

9.  **Double Band Exercises:** Use
    two resistance bands
    simultaneously for exercises
    like squats, deadlifts, or rows.
    This increases the resistance,
    making the exercises more
    challenging and effective for
    muscle growth.

10. **Variable Speed Repetitions:**
    Incorporate changes in
    repetition speed within an
    exercise. For instance, perform

slow and controlled reps, then
switch to fast and explosive
reps. This variation challenges
muscle endurance and power.

Maintain proper form and prioritize
safety when implementing advanced
resistance band techniques. It's
essential to have a good
understanding of your current fitness
level and progressively introduce
these techniques into your routine.
Additionally, listen to your body and
avoid overtraining to prevent injury.
Consult with a fitness professional if
you're unsure about incorporating
advanced techniques into your
resistance band workouts.

# CHAPTER 6

# Tips for Success

## 6.1 Setting Goals

Setting clear and achievable goals is a fundamental step toward success in your resistance band training journey. Well-defined goals can keep you motivated, focused, and on track. Here are some tips for setting goals effectively:

1. **Be Specific:** Define your goals in precise terms. Instead of a vague goal like "get stronger," aim for something specific like "increase my bicep curl resistance by 10 pounds in three months."

2. **Make Them Measurable:**
Ensure your goals are
quantifiable so that you can
track your progress. Use
numbers or metrics to measure
your success. For example,
"perform 15 consecutive push-
ups" is measurable.

3. **Set Realistic Expectations:**
While it's essential to challenge
yourself, be realistic about your
starting point and your potential
for growth. Setting unrealistic
goals can lead to frustration and
burnout.

4. **Set Short-Term and Long-
Term Goals:** Establish both
short-term goals (achievable in
weeks or months) and long-
term goals (six months to a
year). Short-term goals can help
you stay motivated, while long-

term goals provide a broader perspective.

5. **Prioritize Your Goals:** Determine which goals are most important to you and focus on them. Trying to achieve too many goals simultaneously can be overwhelming. Concentrate on the most critical ones first.

6. **Create a Plan:** Develop a structured plan for how you will work toward your goals. Include specific exercises, frequencies, and progress tracking. A well-structured plan increases the likelihood of success.

7. **Set Milestones:** Break your long-term goals into smaller milestones. Each milestone

represents a step closer to your ultimate goal, making it easier to track your progress and stay motivated.

8. **Consider Both Process and Outcome Goals:** Process goals focus on the steps and actions you need to take to achieve your outcome goals. For example, "exercise for 30 minutes five days a week" is a process goal that can lead to achieving an outcome goal like weight loss.

9. **Reevaluate and Adjust:** Regularly review your progress and adjust your goals as needed. If you achieve a goal sooner than expected, set a new one to keep your motivation high.

10. **Share Your Goals:** Consider sharing your goals with a friend, family member, or fitness coach. Having someone to hold you accountable can increase your commitment to your goals.

11. **Stay Positive:** Maintain a positive attitude and focus on your achievements rather than setbacks. Celebrate your successes, no matter how small, and use them as motivation to keep moving forward.

12. **Visualize Success:** Visualize yourself achieving your goals. This mental practice can boost your confidence and motivation.

13. **Stay Flexible:** Life can be unpredictable. Be flexible and

adaptable with your goals. If you encounter obstacles or setbacks, adjust your plan as necessary but stay committed to your overall objective.

14. **Keep a Journal:** Document your progress, workouts, and feelings in a training journal. It can serve as a source of motivation and help you identify what's working and what needs improvement.

Setting well-defined and achievable goals is an essential part of your resistance band training journey. By following these tips, you can create a roadmap to success and stay motivated as you work toward your desired outcomes.

## 6.2 Tracking Your Progress

Monitoring your progress in your resistance band training is crucial for staying motivated, identifying areas for improvement, and reaching your fitness goals. Here are some effective tips for tracking your progress:

1. **Keep a Workout Journal:** Maintain a dedicated journal or digital document where you record each workout session. Include details such as the date, exercises performed, sets, reps, resistance band used, and any notes on how you felt during the workout.

2. **Take Before and After Photos:** Capture photographs of your physique before you start your training and at

regular intervals as you progress. Visual evidence can be a powerful motivator.

3. **Measurements:** Record measurements of key body parts such as your arms, chest, waist, hips, thighs, and calves. Periodically re-measure to track changes in muscle size or fat loss.

4. **Body Weight:** Regularly weigh yourself, preferably at the same time of day and under consistent conditions (e.g., after waking up and using the bathroom). Note any fluctuations in your weight.

5. **Strength Levels:** Keep track of the resistance band color or level used for each exercise. As you progress, you should see an

increase in the resistance level required to maintain the same level of challenge.

6. **Fitness Testing:** Conduct periodic fitness tests to evaluate your strength, endurance, and flexibility. For instance, test your maximum push-ups, plank duration, or squat repetitions to see improvements over time.

7. **Keep a Training Calendar:** Use a calendar or fitness app to schedule your workouts and track your consistency. Check off each workout as you complete it to stay accountable.

8. **Set Benchmark Workouts:** Designate specific workouts as benchmarks that you revisit at regular intervals. Compare your performance in these

benchmark workouts to gauge progress.

9.  **Use Technology:** Many fitness apps and wearable devices can help you track workouts, heart rate, calories burned, and other fitness metrics. These tools can provide valuable data and insights.

10. **Listen to Your Body:** Pay attention to how your body feels during and after workouts. Notice any improvements in energy levels, muscle soreness, or overall well-being.

11. **Diet and Nutrition Tracking:** If your goal involves weight management or improving your diet, consider tracking your food intake and nutritional

choices. Many apps can assist with this.

12. **Reflect on Your Goals:** Regularly review your fitness goals and assess your progress. Make necessary adjustments to your goals or workout routine if needed.

13. **Seek Professional Guidance:** If you're serious about your fitness journey, consider consulting a personal trainer, fitness coach, or physical therapist. They can provide guidance and conduct more advanced assessments of your progress.

14. **Celebrate Achievements:** Acknowledge and celebrate your accomplishments. Whether it's completing a

challenging workout, hitting a new personal record, or achieving a weight loss milestone, celebrate your success.

15. **Stay Consistent:** Consistency is key. Stick to your tracking routines and ensure that you continue to monitor your progress over the long term.

Consistently tracking your progress, you can stay motivated and make informed decisions about adjusting your resistance band training program to align with your fitness goals. Whether you're aiming to build muscle, improve endurance, or enhance flexibility, monitoring your progress is an essential part of your fitness journey.

# 6.3 Overcoming Common Challenges

Resistance band training offers numerous benefits, but like any fitness regimen, it comes with its share of challenges. Here are some common challenges you might face and strategies to overcome them:

1. **Lack of Motivation:**

    - **Solution:** Find your intrinsic motivation by setting clear goals, tracking your progress, and reminding yourself why you started. Consider working out with a friend, following a structured training program, or trying new exercises to keep things interesting.

2. **Plateaus:**

- **Solution:** Change up your routine by introducing new exercises, altering your resistance band levels, incorporating advanced techniques, or focusing on different muscle groups. Plateaus can also indicate the need for rest and recovery.

3. **Resistance Band Wear and Tear:**

- **Solution:** Invest in high-quality resistance bands and handle them with care. Replace bands that show signs of wear, such as small tears or weakened elasticity.

Store them properly, away from direct sunlight or extreme temperatures.

4. **Injury Risk:**

   - **Solution:** Focus on proper form and technique to reduce the risk of injury. Consult with a fitness professional to ensure you're performing exercises correctly. Warm up before your workouts, stretch, and cool down afterward. Listen to your body and avoid overexertion.

5. **Consistency Issues:**

   - **Solution:** Establish a regular workout schedule

and make it a habit. Set reminders or use fitness apps to help you stay consistent. Find a workout time that fits your daily routine and stick to it.

6. **Time Constraints:**

- **Solution:** Opt for shorter, more intense workouts if you have limited time. High-intensity interval training (HIIT) can be very effective and time-efficient. You can also break your workouts into shorter sessions throughout the day if needed.

7. **Boredom:**

- **Solution:** Keep your workouts fresh by trying different exercises, variations, or combining movements. Consider following online workout videos or classes for new ideas. Outdoor workouts or working out in a different environment can also add variety.

8. **Difficulty in Progression:**

    - **Solution:** Gradually increase resistance or intensity as you become stronger. Explore advanced resistance band techniques and focus on progressive overload. Remember that progress may be slow but consistency is key.

9. **Overtraining:**

- **Solution:** Ensure you allow sufficient rest and recovery between workouts. Avoid working the same muscle groups on consecutive days. Pay attention to your body's signals, such as excessive fatigue or persistent soreness, and adjust your training accordingly.

10. **Self-Doubt:**

- **Solution:** Cultivate a positive mindset by celebrating small achievements and staying patient. Surround yourself with a supportive community, whether that's friends, family, or fellow fitness enthusiasts.

## 11. Inadequate Nutrition:

- **Solution:** Proper nutrition is crucial for energy and recovery. Ensure you're consuming a balanced diet that supports your fitness goals. Consult with a nutritionist if needed.

## 12. External Distractions:

- **Solution:** Create a dedicated workout space with minimal distractions. Inform family members or roommates of your workout schedule. Consider using

headphones and
motivational music to
stay focused.

13. **Travel or Lack of Access to a Gym:**

- **Solution:** Resistance bands are portable and easy to carry while traveling. You can continue your workouts in hotel rooms or at home. Many resistance band exercises require minimal space and equipment.

Challenges are a natural part of any fitness journey. It's important to adapt, stay flexible, and keep your goals in mind. With determination and the right strategies, you can overcome these challenges and make progress in your resistance band training.

## 6.4 Embracing a Sustainable Fitness Routine

Creating a sustainable fitness routine with resistance bands involves making choices that are realistic, enjoyable, and maintainable over the long term. Here are some tips to help you build a fitness routine that you can stick with:

1. **Set Realistic Goals:** Establish fitness goals that are achievable and sustainable. This can help prevent burnout and frustration. Consider both short-term and long-term objectives.

2. **Find Activities You Enjoy:** Choose exercises and activities

that you genuinely enjoy. When you like what you're doing, it's easier to stay motivated and consistent.

3.  **Variety and Challenge:** Keep your routine interesting by incorporating a variety of exercises, including resistance band workouts, cardio, flexibility, and balance training. Change your routine regularly to challenge your body and prevent boredom.

4.  **Prioritize Recovery:** Allow your body time to rest and recover. Overtraining can lead to burnout and injuries. Include rest days in your routine, and consider activities like yoga or foam rolling to aid in recovery.

5.  **Consistent Schedule:** Establish a workout schedule that fits your daily routine. Consistency is key to long-term success. Whether it's morning, noon, or evening, stick to a regular exercise time.

6.  **Listen to Your Body:** Pay attention to how your body feels. If you're fatigued, sore, or injured, it's okay to take a break or modify your workouts. Be kind to yourself and adapt your routine as needed.

7.  **Set Achievable Milestones:** Celebrate your accomplishments, no matter how small they may seem. Acknowledge your progress to stay motivated and boost your self-confidence.

8. **Build a Support System:**
   Share your fitness journey with friends, family, or fellow fitness enthusiasts. A support system can provide encouragement and accountability.

9. **Nutrition and Hydration:**
   Fuel your body with proper nutrition and stay hydrated. A balanced diet is essential for sustaining your fitness routine. Consult with a nutritionist if needed.

10. **Revisit and Adjust:**
   Periodically review your goals and assess your fitness routine. Make adjustments based on your progress and changing needs. Your routine should evolve with you.

11. **Use Technology:** Fitness apps, wearable devices, and online communities can help you stay motivated and track your progress. Consider using these tools to enhance your routine.

12. **Consult a Professional:** If you're unsure about your routine, consider consulting a fitness professional or personal trainer. They can provide guidance, tailored programs, and ensure you're exercising safely and effectively.

13. **Maintain a Positive Mindset:** Focus on the positive aspects of your fitness journey. Embrace challenges as opportunities for growth, and don't let setbacks deter you from your long-term goals.

14. **Include Rest and Recovery:**
    Rest is a critical component of
    any sustainable fitness routine.
    Ensure you get enough sleep,
    and prioritize active recovery
    techniques like stretching, foam
    rolling, and mobility exercises.

15. **Set Lifetime Goals:** Consider
    what you want to achieve in the
    long run, not just in the short
    term. Sustainable fitness is a
    lifelong commitment to health
    and well-being.

Embracing a sustainable fitness
routine with resistance bands means
making fitness a part of your daily
life, enjoying the journey, and staying
committed to your long-term health
and fitness goals. Remember that the
key to success is finding a balance
that works for you and makes exercise

a sustainable and enjoyable aspect of
your life.